HOLISTIC APPROACHES TO HEALING CHILDHOOD

Holistic Strategies for Nurturing Childhood Well-Being and Fostering Emotional Healing

DR. CHRIS FRIEDRICH

Disclaimer

This book on Herbal Remedies is intended solely for informational and educational purposes.

The content provided within this book is based on general knowledge and should not be considered as professional advice. The author is not a licensed medical professional, and the information presented here is not intended to diagnose, treat, cure, or prevent any disease.

Readers are advised to consult with qualified healthcare professionals before initiating any herbal remedies or making changes to their existing health regimen. The author and publisher disclaim any responsibility for any adverse effects or consequences resulting from the use of information contained in this book.

It's important to note that the content of this book is not endorsed by any specific platform or affiliated with any product or service.

The author does not receive any compensation or benefits from the promotion of specific herbal products or brands.

Readers should exercise their discretion and judgment when applying the information from this book, and they are encouraged to conduct further research and seek guidance from healthcare professionals to make informed decisions about their health and well-being.

The book "Holistic Approaches to Healing Childhood Trauma" is a significant addition to the fields of mental health and child development. It offers a thorough examination of the various aspects linked to childhood trauma as well as creative approaches to holistic healing. The book is organized methodically, starting with an introduction that defines childhood trauma, clarifies the goal of the work, and emphasizes the value of holistic approaches in resolving this complicated problem.

The first chapter of the book explores the intricacies of childhood trauma, explaining the different forms that include physical abuse, emotional abuse, neglect, sexual abuse, and witnessing violence. It also carefully looks at the long-term consequences of childhood trauma, including the effects on physical health, emotional and psychological effects, and the complex interactions with interpersonal relationships.

A thorough definition of holistic healing, an examination of various holistic modalities (such as the mind-body connection, spirituality in healing, and integrative therapies), and an emphasis on the value of a thorough assessment, resilience factors assessment, and identification of trauma triggers are all covered in detail in Chapter 2.

Turning now to Chapter 3, the book delves into therapeutic modalities, including art therapy, animal-assisted therapy, and yoga in addition to more conventional psychotherapy approaches like cognitive-behavioral therapy (CBT) and eye movement desensitization and reprocessing (EMDR). Each modality is analyzed in light of how well it works for treating childhood trauma.

The book emphasizes the value of support networks, safe spaces, dietary considerations, physical activity, and a variety of self-care techniques. Chapters 4 through 7 walk readers through the establishment of nurturing environments, nutritional and physical well-being, and holistic self-care practices. It also incorporates cultural and spiritual perspectives into the healing process, recognizing the importance of cultural sensitivity and spiritual approaches in fostering recovery.

The book's last chapter covers prevention and community outreach strategies, emphasizing community-based education and advocacy, early intervention approaches, and school-based prevention programs. It also stresses the significance of identifying at-risk children, putting school-based prevention programs into place, and creating trauma-informed communities.

Essentially, "Holistic Approaches to Healing Childhood Trauma" broadens the scholarly conversation about childhood trauma while also offering practitioners, educators, and caregivers a useful manual for holistic healing techniques. This book serves as a lighthouse of knowledge and direction, bridging the knowledge gap between theory and practical solutions, ultimately enhancing the resilience and well-being of traumatized children.

Overview

A comprehensive understanding of the complexities involved in the healing process can be established by delving into the purpose of the book, defining childhood trauma, and emphasizing the importance of holistic approaches. Childhood trauma is a pervasive issue that can have profound and lasting impacts on an individual's mental, emotional, and physical well-being. As society becomes more aware of the prevalence and severity of childhood trauma, there is a growing need for effective approaches to healing and recovery.

The Book's Objective

This book's main goal is to provide a thorough resource for mental health professionals, educators, caregivers, and anyone else who wants to learn more about the complex nature of childhood trauma and address it. It also aims to close the knowledge gap between theory and practice by providing insights into evidence-based holistic interventions that cover the psychological, emotional, social, and physical aspects of healing. Finally, by examining a variety of therapeutic modalities and cutting-edge interventions, the book hopes to add to the body of knowledge that supports more complex and effective approaches to healing childhood trauma.

Definition Of Trauma In Childhood

To effectively tailor holistic interventions that address each individual's unique needs, it is imperative to first establish a clear understanding of what is meant by childhood trauma, which is defined as experiences that pose a significant threat to a child's physical or emotional well-being. Childhood trauma can take many different forms, such as physical, emotional, or sexual abuse, neglect, witnessing domestic violence, or exposure to other traumatic events. The impact of childhood trauma extends beyond the immediate experience, often shaping an individual's cognitive and emotional development, interpersonal relationships, and overall mental health.

Importance Of Holistic Methods

Because the mind, body, and spirit are interconnected, holistic approaches to healing childhood trauma take into account the whole person, as opposed to traditional therapeutic methods that might only address cognitive or behavioral aspects.

Taking a holistic approach is important because it can address the intricate interplay of factors that contribute to trauma and its aftermath.

Holistic approaches include expressive arts, mindfulness practices, psychological therapies, somatic interventions, and nutritional support, among other modalities. By addressing the emotional, physical, and spiritual dimensions simultaneously, holistic approaches aim to facilitate comprehensive healing, build resilience, and promote long-term well-being.

Psychotherapy's Place In Holistic Healing

A fundamental component of holistic approaches to healing childhood trauma is psychotherapy, which offers a regulated and nurturing space for people to examine and work through their traumatic experiences. Different therapeutic modalities, including dialectical behavior therapy (DBT), psychodynamic therapy, and cognitive-behavioral therapy (CBT), can be incorporated into a holistic framework to assist people in recognizing and reframing maladaptive thought patterns, controlling their emotions, and developing more healthy coping mechanisms. Additionally, trauma-informed psychotherapy places special emphasis on establishing a safe therapeutic alliance, acknowledging the personal impact of trauma, and encouraging a collaborative and empowering healing process.

Somatic Experiencing's Place In Holistic Healing

Developed by Dr. Peter A. Levine, somatic experiencing is an essential part of holistic approaches to healing childhood trauma.

It acknowledges the physiological and nervous system reactions to trauma and focuses on reestablishing balance in the autonomic nervous system, which may become dysregulated after trauma. By combining body awareness, mindfulness, and gradual exposure, somatic experiencing enables people to release stored tension and stress in their bodies. By addressing the somatic aspects of trauma, this approach offers an embodied and comprehensive healing path that complements traditional psychotherapy.

The Combination Of Therapies With Expressive Arts

The inclusion of expressive arts therapies in a holistic approach recognizes the variety of ways in which individuals can interact with their healing journey. Art therapy, music therapy, and dance/movement therapy are examples of modalities that play a crucial role in holistic healing.

These therapies offer non-verbal avenues for individuals to express and process their emotions, avoiding potential language barriers that may impede traditional talk therapy. The creative and symbolic nature of expressive arts allows for the exploration of trauma in a safe and empowering way. Artistically expressing oneself can lead to self-discovery, encourage emotional regulation, and improve the integration of disparate aspects of the self.

Holistic Healing And Mindfulness

Through the cultivation of present-moment awareness without judgment, mindfulness practices—which include breathing exercises, body scans, and meditation—can help people become more aware of their inner experiences. Mindfulness increases people's ability to tolerate discomfort, control their emotions, and create a sense of safety within themselves. It also plays a significant role in lowering symptoms of anxiety, depression, and post-traumatic stress disorder, making it an invaluable tool in the holistic toolbox for healing childhood trauma.

The Value Of Relationships And Social Support

Social support acts as a buffer against the negative effects of trauma and contributes to an individual's sense of belonging and safety. Holistic approaches emphasize the importance of cultivating a supportive network of family, friends, and community.

Group therapy, peer support, and community-based initiatives contribute to a sense of collective healing, reducing isolation, and fostering resilience in the face of adversity. Holistic healing goes beyond individual therapeutic interventions to include the broader context of social support and connection.

Nutritional Guidance For Comprehensive Health

A growing body of research indicates that diet can affect mood, cognition, and overall mental well-being. Including a nutrition-focused approach entails addressing potential nutritional deficiencies, taking into account the impact of diet on inflammation and gut health, and acknowledging the role of specific nutrients in supporting the nervous system. By incorporating nutritional support into holistic interventions, practitioners aim to optimize the physiological foundation for mental and emotional well-being, promoting a holistic approach to healing.

The relationship between nutrition and mental health is a burgeoning area of research within the holistic healing paradigm.

Finally, holistic approaches to healing childhood trauma provide an integrative and multifaceted framework that acknowledges the interdependence of the mind, body, and spirit. This book has defined childhood trauma, explored the rationale behind exploring holistic approaches, and emphasized the need to implement comprehensive strategies in addressing the intricate effects of early adverse experiences.

From expressive arts therapies and psychotherapy to mindfulness practices, social support, and nutritional interventions, holistic approaches encompass a wide range of modalities aimed at promoting holistic well-being. By appreciating and embracing the richness of holistic healing, we clear the way for a more compassionate and successful response to the intricacies of childhood trauma.

CHAPTER ONE
UNDERSTANDING CHILDHOOD TRAUMA

A person's physical, emotional, and psychological development can be greatly impacted by a variety of traumatic experiences that occur during childhood. Childhood trauma is a pervasive and complex issue that can have profound and long-lasting effects on an individual's well-being.

It is important to identify and comprehend the different types of childhood trauma to develop effective holistic approaches to healing. These forms of trauma include physical abuse, emotional abuse, neglect, sexual abuse, and witnessing violence.

Kinds Of Trauma In Childhood:

<u>Physical Maltreatment:</u>

Physical abuse occurs when a caregiver intentionally causes harm or injury to a child.

This can include hitting, kicking, slapping, or any other type of physical aggression. While bruises, broken bones, or other visible injuries can be the immediate result of physical abuse, there are long-term effects that go beyond the physical realm and negatively impact a child's mental and emotional health.

<u>Abuse of Emotions:</u>

In contrast to physical abuse, emotional abuse may not always be evident, making it difficult to identify. However, the emotional wounds inflicted during childhood can have long-lasting effects on an individual's mental health and self-esteem. Emotional abuse is defined by persistent verbal or non-verbal behaviors that belittle a child's sense of self-worth and emotional well-being. It can involve constant criticism, humiliation, or rejection.

Ignorance:

For a child to develop healthily, caregivers must give them the care, attention, and supervision they need. This can include emotional and physical neglect, which includes depriving a child of love, affection, and emotional support, as well as inadequate nutrition or medical attention.

Neglect can impede a child's cognitive, social, and emotional growth, which can result in a variety of difficulties as they grow older.

Sexual Mistreatment:

Any non-consensual sexual activity imposed on a child is considered sexual abuse. This can include rape, molestation, or exposure to explicit materials. Sexual abuse has a profound psychological impact on a child, causing emotional trauma, feelings of guilt and shame, and distorted perceptions of intimacy and relationships. These effects can last into adulthood and negatively impact the individual's ability to form healthy connections.

Observing acts of violence:

Children who witness violence—whether it be in the form of community violence or domestic violence between caregivers—experience trauma indirectly. This type of trauma is frequently linked to a variety of behavioral and emotional problems, such as anxiety, depression, and aggression. Witnessing violence can create a pervasive sense of fear and insecurity, affecting a child's sense of safety and trust.

Effects Of Childhood Trauma In The Long Run

Physical Health Repercussions:

Beyond its effects on the emotional and psychological domain, childhood trauma also has an impact on physical health. Research has linked childhood trauma to several health problems, such as autoimmune disorders, chronic pain, and cardiovascular diseases. The stress response that is triggered by childhood trauma can result in long-term physiological changes, which increase the likelihood of physical health problems in adulthood.

<u>Impact on Emotion and Psychology:</u>

Individuals who have experienced trauma may struggle with mental health issues like anxiety, depression, post-traumatic stress disorder (PTSD), and substance abuse. The emotional scars left by childhood trauma can impact self-esteem, identity formation, and the ability to cope with life's challenges. Childhood trauma can have profound and lasting effects on emotional and psychological well-being.

Effect On Relationships With Others:

Childhood trauma has important relational ramifications that impact an individual's capacity to establish and sustain healthy relationships. Survivors of childhood trauma frequently struggle with trust issues, feelings of abandonment, and communication breakdowns.

These relational patterns can impact friendships, romantic relationships, and professional collaborations.

Holistic Methods For Resolving Trauma In Childhood:

Holistic approaches to healing childhood trauma acknowledge the connection between physical, emotional, and psychological health. They go beyond conventional therapeutic techniques, combining different modalities to address the complex nature of trauma. Holistic healing acknowledges the need for a thorough and customized treatment plan, taking into account the individual experiences and difficulties that each survivor faces.

Interventions Therapeutic:

Holistic approaches to healing childhood trauma heavily emphasize therapeutic interventions. Therapies that focus on the emotional and psychological effects of trauma, such as Trauma-Focused Cognitive Behavioral Therapy (TF-CBT) and Eye Movement Desensitization and Reprocessing (EMDR), give survivors the tools they need to process their experiences, manage their symptoms, and create healthier coping mechanisms.

Mind-Body Methods:

The field of holistic healing acknowledges the complex relationship between the mind and body and highlights the role that mind-body therapies play in the healing process. Holistic healing practices include yoga, meditation, and mindfulness, which all help to promote relaxation, self-awareness, and emotional regulation. By addressing the mental and physical aspects of trauma, these practices also support the general well-being of survivors.

Therapies in the Creative Arts:

These nonverbal outlets for self-expression allow individuals to explore and communicate their experiences in ways that may be difficult through traditional talk therapy. Creative arts therapies, such as art therapy, music therapy, and dance/movement therapy, offer alternative avenues for survivors to express and process their emotions. Creative arts therapies can be especially helpful for those who find it difficult to articulate their emotions verbally.

Somatic Awareness:

To release the physical manifestations of trauma, survivors can learn to regulate their nervous system responses and release stored tension and stress through guided awareness of bodily sensations. Somatic experiencing is particularly helpful for individuals with complex trauma and dissociation. It acknowledges that trauma is retained in the body in addition to the mind. Changes to a Holistic Lifestyle:

Beyond therapeutic interventions, holistic healing encompasses lifestyle modifications that support overall well-being.

These include stress management, exercise, proper diet, and sleep. A healthy lifestyle builds emotional stability, physical resilience, and improved cognitive function—all of which serve as strong foundations for the healing process.

Social and Community Support:

A supportive network of friends, family, and community resources can give survivors a sense of belonging and validation. Peer support groups, community organizations, and advocacy efforts contribute to creating a supportive environment for individuals on their healing journey. Holistic approaches recognize the social dimension of trauma and emphasize the importance of community and social support.

<u>Diversity and Cultural Competence:</u>

Culturally competent and diverse approaches to healing childhood trauma are prioritized because they recognize that people with diverse cultural backgrounds may have particular needs and perspectives. Culturally sensitive interventions guarantee that survivors receive treatment that honors their cultural identity, values, and beliefs. By adjusting interventions to the individual's cultural context, this inclusivity increases the efficacy of holistic healing.

<u>Prevention and Education:</u>

Holistic approaches place a strong emphasis on education and prevention initiatives in addition to therapeutic interventions for trauma survivors.

Educating the public about the prevalence and effects of childhood trauma, offering guidance on healthy parenting techniques, and supporting laws that promote children's well-being all help to reduce the likelihood of future traumas. By addressing the underlying causes of trauma, holistic approaches aim to build a society that is more resilient and supportive for coming generations.

By addressing the various and long-lasting effects of trauma, holistic approaches to healing childhood trauma aim to provide survivors with comprehensive and individualized support. Through therapeutic interventions, mind-body approaches, creative arts therapies, somatic experiences, lifestyle changes, and community support, these approaches recognize the complex interplay between physical, emotional, and psychological well-being.

CHAPTER 2
FRAMEWORK FOR HOLISTIC HEALING

A multifaceted approach is necessary for effective recovery from childhood trauma. Holistic healing is a comprehensive approach that takes into account the interconnectedness of various aspects of an individual's well-being, including physical, mental, emotional, and spiritual. It emphasizes the importance of treating the underlying causes of trauma rather than just treating its symptoms and integrates various therapeutic modalities, acknowledging the synergy between the mind, body, and spirit.

Holistic Methods For Treating Childhood Trauma

Holistic healing defined

In the context of childhood trauma, holistic healing entails a paradigm shift from a reductionist approach to a more inclusive perspective. It includes a variety of interventions that address the underlying emotional and psychological imbalances as well as the visible symptoms of trauma. This approach recognizes the dynamic interplay between an individual's physical, mental, and spiritual aspects, acknowledging that true healing necessitates attention to all dimensions of the self. By fostering self-awareness and agency, holistic healing empowers individuals to take an active role in their recovery.

Holistic Methods For Treating Childhood Trauma

Mind-Body Link

The mind-body connection is a cornerstone of holistic healing when it comes to childhood trauma. It highlights the reciprocal relationship between mental and physical health, emphasizing the necessity of addressing both at the same time. Practices like mindfulness, yoga, and somatic experiencing are essential parts of the mind-body connection, assisting people in regulating their emotions, lowering their stress levels, and reestablishing a connection with their bodies. By recognizing and fostering this connection, holistic approaches seek to promote overall well-being and restore equilibrium.

Spirituality in Medical Practice

Integrating spirituality into the healing process acknowledges the existential aspects of trauma and promotes a holistic understanding of one's life journey. Spirituality plays a significant role in holistic approaches to healing childhood trauma. It is not necessarily limited to religious beliefs but encompasses a broader sense of meaning, purpose, and connection to something beyond oneself. Spiritual practices, such as meditation, prayer, and reflection, give individuals tools to explore and understand the deeper dimensions of their trauma. This exploration can lead to a sense of transcendence, which can help with resilience and a renewed sense of hope.

<u>Complementary Medicine</u>

To address the complexity of childhood trauma, holistic healing integrates a variety of therapeutic modalities, including energy healing, massage, acupuncture, and cognitive-behavioral therapies. This integration acknowledges that people respond differently to different interventions and that a customized, all-encompassing treatment plan is necessary. Holistic approaches offer a more individualized and successful route to healing by fusing evidence-based practices with alternative therapies.

Value Of A Comprehensive Evaluation

<u>Finding the Triggers of Trauma</u>

A thorough evaluation that pinpoints trauma triggers—which can be situational, emotional, or sensory—is an essential part of holistic healing. Holistic assessments go beyond standard diagnostic criteria to explore the particular situations and stimuli that cause traumatic reactions. With this level of detail, therapists can create targeted interventions, like desensitization or exposure therapy, to progressively lessen the impact of triggers and improve a person's coping mechanisms.

<u>Evaluating Resilience Elements</u>

Comprehensive assessments look at things like social support, coping mechanisms, and positive relationships that contribute to an individual's resilience. By emphasizing these strengths, holistic healing encourages the development of a positive self-concept and gives people the confidence to navigate the healing process. Holistic approaches emphasize the importance of not only identifying trauma-related challenges but also assessing an individual's resilience factors. Resilience involves the capacity to adapt and bounce back from adversity, and recognizing these inherent strengths is vital for effective intervention.

Ultimately, the goal of holistic healing is not only to alleviate symptoms but also to foster resilience, self-awareness, and a sense of empowerment in individuals on their journey toward recovery. Holistic healing offers a comprehensive and interconnected framework for addressing childhood trauma. It recognizes the complex relationship between the mind, body, and spirit and incorporates diverse therapeutic modalities to acknowledge the complexity of trauma and tailor interventions to the individual. The emphasis on comprehensive assessment, including the identification of trauma triggers and assessment of resilience factors, ensures a targeted and successful healing process.

CHAPTER THREE
THERAPEUTIC MODALITIES

A person's well-being can be significantly impacted by childhood trauma, which can have a long-lasting effect on many aspects of their life. When it comes to treating childhood trauma, a holistic approach is frequently thought to be necessary. This entails incorporating therapeutic modalities that address the emotional, cognitive, and physical aspects of a person's experience. Of the many therapeutic modalities available, psychotherapy is crucial because it offers a safe and structured space for people to process and examine their traumatic experiences.

In the field of psychotherapy, Cognitive-Behavioral Therapy (CBT) is a popular and scientifically validated method that emphasizes the interaction between thoughts, feelings, and behaviors to recognize and alter maladaptive patterns. When it comes to childhood trauma, CBT assists clients in identifying and disputing the negative thought patterns that are connected to their traumatic experiences, which promotes more positive cognitive and affective reactions.

An additional notable psychotherapy technique is Eye Movement Desensitization and Reprocessing (EMDR), which works especially well for trauma patients by helping them process upsetting memories. Based on the theory that bilateral stimulation, like guided eye movements, can help the brain integrate and process traumatic experiences, EMDR uses an eight-phase structured approach to help patients reprocess traumatic memories, lessening their emotional impact and promoting adaptive resolution.

Play Therapy is a valuable adjunct to traditional talk therapies in the holistic healing of childhood trauma. It acknowledges that children find it easier to express themselves through play than through verbal communication, and it uses a variety of play-based techniques to support children in exploring and communicating their feelings, ideas, and experiences in a way that is non-threatening and developmentally appropriate.

Outside of traditional psychotherapy, alternative therapies are important because they provide a variety of pathways for the healing of childhood trauma. For example, art therapy uses the creative process to facilitate emotional processing and self-expression. Through artistic expression, patients can externalize their inner experiences, giving therapists important insights into their feelings and perceptions. This modality is especially helpful for people who have difficulty expressing themselves verbally.

Another approach that utilizes the therapeutic benefits of human-animal interactions is called "animal-assisted therapy," in which animals— typically horses or dogs—are incorporated into the therapeutic process to improve emotional well-being and offer a sense of security and support. The nonjudgmental and unconditional acceptance of animals can form a special therapeutic bond that promotes trust and allows for the expression of emotions, particularly in people who may find it difficult to form interpersonal relationships.

Yoga and Mindfulness Practices: With their emphasis on breath, movement, and meditation, yoga can help regulate the nervous system, reduce anxiety, and improve overall emotional resilience. Mindfulness practices, on the other hand, like meditation, cultivate awareness and acceptance, empowering people to approach their traumatic experiences with a non-judgmental and compassionate mindset. Together, these practices emphasize the mind-body connection and encourage individuals to be present in the moment.

a comprehensive integration of therapeutic modalities that address the complex aspects of the individual's experience is necessary for a holistic approach to healing childhood trauma. Psychotherapeutic modalities such as CBT and

EMDR offer structured frameworks for cognitive and emotional processing, while Play Therapy acknowledges the special needs of children in self-expression. Alternative therapies such as Art Therapy, Animal-Assisted Therapy, and Yoga with Mindfulness Practices provide a variety of opportunities for self-expression, emotional regulation, and holistic well-being. By integrating these approaches, therapists can customize interventions to the specific needs of each individual, promoting a thorough and successful healing process for childhood trauma.

CHAPTER 4
DEVELOPING A SUPPORTIVE ENVIRONMENT

The development and maintenance of a caring and supportive environment is essential to the holistic approach to healing childhood trauma. It involves several factors, all of which have a substantial impact on the general health of a traumatized child. Among the main ones is the establishment of a strong support network, which includes social relationships, family dynamics, and community involvement.

A supportive and compassionate family environment can provide traumatized children with the emotional scaffolding they need to feel secure and like they belong. The value of a support system in the healing of childhood trauma cannot be overstated. Family dynamics, as a subset of this support system, become a critical factor. It involves understanding the intricate relationships within a family and their impact on the child's healing process.

For a child recovering from trauma, having positive and stable social relationships can act as a buffer against the negative effects of the traumatic experience. Friends, mentors, and other positive influences contribute to a child's sense of identity and self-worth. Humans are inherently social creatures, and the quality of social interactions has a profound effect on mental and emotional well-being.

Collaboration between schools, families, and the community creates a holistic and comprehensive support structure. School and community involvement expands the support system further. Schools can function as both educational institutions and environments that foster emotional and social development. Teachers and school staff are essential in identifying and meeting the needs of traumatized children. Community involvement broadens the support network by offering additional resources and perspectives that aid in the healing process of the child.

Establishing Safe Areas:

The idea of creating safe spaces is central to the holistic approach to healing childhood trauma. Safe spaces are environments that are both physical and emotional that support a child's healing and development. This includes making sure that homes and schools are safe and meeting the unique needs of traumatized children.

Establishing a predictable, stable, and nurturing home environment is essential to the healing process for traumatized children, who frequently experience elevated levels of anxiety and fear. Family members and caregivers are vital in creating this sense of safety, which is largely dependent on open communication, regular routines, and the provision of emotional support.

Educational settings, such as classrooms and schools, are crucial to the healing process because they can either exacerbate or lessen the distress experienced by traumatized children. Establishing safe spaces for learning entails incorporating trauma-informed practices into the educational system and training teachers to identify and address the special needs of traumatized students. These needs might include reducing triggers, offering extra support, and cultivating an environment of understanding and empathy within the school community.

The establishment of safe spaces, in summary, is essential to a holistic approach to healing childhood trauma. By addressing the psychological and physical dimensions of safety, caregivers, educators, and communities can make a substantial positive impact on the general well-being of traumatized children. This approach acknowledges that safety is not only a fundamental need but also a cornerstone of the child's path to recovery and resilience.

CHAPTER 5
HYGIENIC AND PHYSICAL SUMMARY

Childhood trauma can have significant and lasting effects on mental health, so taking a holistic approach to healing means taking into account the importance of both physical and nutritional well-being. One important component of this approach is the impact of nutrition on mental health, as new research is illuminating the complex relationship between our diet and brain function.

Foods that boost the brain, like those high in antioxidants, omega-3 fatty acids, and essential vitamins, are critical for supporting cognitive functions and reducing the effects of trauma. Knowing the unique nutritional requirements of those who have experienced childhood trauma becomes crucial for creating effective interventions.

Going deeper into the nutritional side, it is imperative to investigate dietary guidelines specific to the healing of childhood trauma. Since malnourishment can worsen mental health issues, trauma specialists need to stress the importance of a balanced diet that meets the special needs of trauma survivors. Sufficient consumption of nutrients such as B vitamins, magnesium, and amino acids becomes critical because these nutrients are linked to the production of neurotransmitters and general brain health. By incorporating nutritional counseling and education into therapeutic interventions, individuals can be empowered to make decisions about their diet, fostering a healing environment.

Including physical activity in the holistic approach is another essential component. Regular exercise has been shown to alleviate symptoms of anxiety and depression, which are common comorbidities among trauma survivors. Exercise is also known to be a stress reliever, and its benefits can be extended to those who are coping with the aftermath of childhood trauma. Professionals can effectively tailor interventions by knowing the physiological and psychological mechanisms that underlie the positive effects of exercise on mental health.

The integration of yoga and movement therapies into trauma-informed care broadens the spectrum of available interventions by acknowledging the diversity of individual preferences and responses to different modalities. Yoga and movement therapies are specialized forms of physical activity that have gained prominence in the holistic healing of childhood trauma. These practices incorporate mindfulness, breathing techniques, and intentional movement, going beyond conventional exercise. The mind-body connection inherent in yoga and movement therapies offers trauma survivors a unique avenue for processing and releasing stored trauma. Research suggests that these practices can contribute to emotional regulation, improved self-awareness, and a sense of empowerment.

 a comprehensive approach to healing childhood trauma entails taking into account both physical and nutritional well-being. Since nutrition has a significant impact on mental health, mental health professionals need to highlight foods that boost the brain and customize dietary recommendations to meet the unique needs of trauma survivors. Moreover, physical activity, including both general exercise and specialized practices like yoga, plays a major role in stress relief and emotional regulation. By combining these factors into therapeutic interventions, a more nuanced and successful approach to healing childhood trauma can be achieved.

CHAPTER 6
HOLISTIC SELF-CARE PRACTICES

A broad range of strategies that take into account the interdependence of the mind, body, and spirit are included in holistic approaches to healing childhood trauma. One important aspect of these approaches is holistic self-care, which acknowledges the importance of promoting one's overall well-being to facilitate healing.

In this investigation, we explore the profound effects of mind-body techniques, including breathing exercises, meditation, and mindfulness. We also look at the therapeutic benefits of journaling and expressive writing, as well as journal prompts that are specifically designed to aid in the healing process.

Mind-body techniques are a cornerstone of holistic approaches to healing childhood trauma.

Two particularly effective methods for fostering a profound sense of awareness and presence are meditation and mindfulness. Drawing from ancient contemplative traditions, meditation involves intentionally cultivating a quiet and focused mind. In addition to being a valuable tool for trauma recovery, mindfulness emphasizes being fully present in the moment. Through mindfulness, people can develop a non-judgmental awareness of their thoughts and emotions, which helps them navigate traumatic experiences with greater resilience.

In the context of trauma healing, breathing exercises are another crucial element of mind-body techniques. Since the breath is so closely linked to emotional states, it becomes an effective means of controlling the nervous system. Methods like diaphragmatic breathing, box breathing, and paced respiration provide people with concrete tools to modify their physiological reactions to stress. Through deliberate and controlled breathing, people can activate the parasympathetic nervous system, which promotes relaxation and counteracts the hyperarousal that is frequently associated with trauma.

Writing can help people externalize and make sense of their experiences. It can also help people organize disorganized thoughts and emotions and gain a deeper understanding of themselves. Writing can be especially cathartic as it can help people release pent-up emotions and gain clarity on their narratives. Journaling and expressive writing are two powerful tools for helping people reflect on and process their feelings as they work through healing from childhood trauma.

The Psychological Benefits of Writing: The cathartic process of writing about emotions helps people confront and reframe their traumatic narratives, fostering a sense of agency and empowerment over their own stories.

Writing about emotions has been shown to have tangible psychological benefits beyond the act of documenting experiences.

One such benefit is that writing about emotions can improve mood, reduce symptoms of anxiety and depression, and improve overall well-being.

By working with these prompts, people can navigate the complexities of their trauma and gradually integrate their experiences into a coherent narrative that supports healing and resilience.

Journal Prompts for Healing are specifically designed to encourage people to explore particular aspects of their experiences, emotions, and beliefs. For example, people may be encouraged to consider the impact of traumatic events on their relationships, worldview, or sense of self.

holistic approaches to healing childhood trauma highlight the connection between mind, body, and spirit. Mind-body practices like breathing exercises, meditation, and mindfulness offer useful tools for controlling the body's emotional and physiological reactions to trauma. Journaling and expressive writing, with their therapeutic advantages and specific prompts, offer spaces for introspection and the reclaiming of one's story. When people practice holistic self-care, they start a healing journey that affects every part of their being and builds resilience and empowerment in the wake of childhood trauma.

CHAPTER 7
INTEGRATING SPIRITUAL AND CULTURAL PERSPECTIVES IS COVERED

A thorough and nuanced approach to healing childhood trauma requires integrating spiritual and cultural perspectives, which is a crucial component of the approach. Understanding the importance of cultural factors is necessary to provide effective healing strategies.

Cultural sensitivity in healing entails understanding diverse cultural backgrounds and acknowledging the impact of cultural norms, values, and traditions on an individual's experience of trauma. Therapists must be aware of cultural nuances to ensure that interventions are respectful of each individual's unique needs.

This cultural sensitivity goes beyond awareness to include adapting therapeutic techniques to fit cultural contexts.

The concept of Understanding Cultural Trauma is an important one to explore within the framework of cultural sensitivity. It entails identifying the collective experiences of particular communities or groups that may contribute to the trauma experienced by individuals within those communities.

By acknowledging historical and cultural factors, therapists can gain a deeper understanding of the causes of trauma, which can lead to more effective interventions. The ultimate goal is to create a safe and compassionate space where individuals can process the complex interactions between personal and collective trauma.

In addition to cultural sensitivity, there is also the idea of Culturally Competent Therapies, which highlights the need for therapists to be knowledgeable about different cultural frameworks and skilled at modifying therapeutic interventions by those frameworks.

Culturally competent therapies aim to actively engage with the client's cultural background, which may entail incorporating cultural rituals, traditions, or storytelling into therapeutic practices to promote a more comprehensive and culturally relevant healing process.

Beyond cultural boundaries, the incorporation of spiritual viewpoints is essential to the comprehensive recovery from childhood trauma. Spiritual Approaches to Healing acknowledge the inherent relationship between spirituality and psychological health.

The foundation of spiritual healing is the discovery of meaning and purpose; therapists support clients in delving into the more profound existential questions associated with their trauma, assisting them in finding purpose in the face of hardship.

This approach is consistent with existential and logotherapy principles, highlighting the potential role that a sense of purpose can play in helping clients overcome trauma.

Incorporating spiritual practices (such as mindfulness, meditation, prayer, or other contemplative practices with spiritual significance) into the therapeutic process is a crucial component of spiritual approaches.

These practices give people tools to connect with their inner selves, which promotes resilience and tranquility. Therapists who integrate spirituality into the healing process recognize and take advantage of the profound effects that spiritual beliefs and practices can have on a patient's path to recovery.

Together, these perspectives contribute to a more comprehensive and effective framework for addressing the complex and deeply rooted effects of childhood trauma. In conclusion, the integration of cultural and spiritual perspectives in healing childhood trauma reflects a holistic understanding of the individual's experience. Cultural sensitivity ensures that therapeutic interventions are tailored to the unique needs of diverse individuals. Spiritual approaches explore the existential and transcendent aspects of healing.

CHAPTER 8
COMMUNITY OUTREACH AND PREVENTION

A comprehensive approach to healing must include both community outreach and childhood trauma prevention. Through proactive measures, society can address the underlying causes of trauma and establish a nurturing environment in which children can flourish. Early intervention strategies are essential to this strategy, with a particular focus on identifying children who are at risk and putting school-based prevention programs into place.

Early Intervention Techniques

In the context of preventing childhood trauma, one of the most important aspects of early intervention is identifying at-risk children. Educators, healthcare providers, and social workers are among the professionals who are essential in identifying signs of distress or vulnerability in children. This requires an understanding of risk factors, which include family dynamics, socioeconomic conditions, and exposure to violence. By identifying at-risk children early on, interventions can be customized to meet their unique needs and prevent the trauma from escalating.

By incorporating prevention efforts into the educational system, society can address trauma at its source and lay the groundwork for healthier development. School-Based Prevention Programs play a significant role in creating a safe and nurturing environment for children.

They can involve a variety of components, including mental health education, conflict resolution training, and fostering positive relationships. Moreover, the implementation of trauma-informed practices within schools can improve teachers' capacity to identify and assist traumatized students.

Advocacy And Community Education

Dispelling myths about trauma, mental health, and the effects of childhood adversity is crucial, and communities can play a key role in reducing the stigma associated with seeking support for trauma-related issues. Reducing stigma is a critical component of community education and advocacy in the context of childhood trauma. Stigmatization can exacerbate the challenges faced by traumatized individuals, preventing them from seeking help or disclosing their experiences.

Encouraging trauma-informed communities means establishing settings that acknowledge and address the effects of trauma on individuals.

This strategy goes beyond individual treatments and aims to turn entire communities into places of support and empathy. Educating community members, such as law enforcement, healthcare professionals, and leaders, about trauma-informed practices can result in a more sympathetic response to trauma survivors. Establishing support networks within communities can also boost resilience and aid in the healing process.

By identifying at-risk children, putting school-based prevention programs into place, lowering stigma, and encouraging trauma-informed communities, society can create a supportive framework for healing and resilience. It is through these comprehensive efforts that we can address the underlying causes of childhood trauma and pave the way for healthier and more resilient future generations. A holistic approach to healing childhood trauma requires a multifaceted strategy that encompasses prevention, early intervention, and community education.

Summary Of Holistic Methods:

When exploring the field of holistic approaches to healing childhood trauma, it is necessary to comprehend the complex ways in which these approaches operate. Holistic healing recognizes that trauma can appear in different aspects of a child's existence. One common method is psychotherapy, in which the child participates in a therapeutic conversation to examine and process traumatic experiences. Cognitive-behavioral therapy (CBT) and dialectical behavior therapy (DBT) are commonly used in this setting to improve negative thought patterns and improve emotional regulation. In addition to traditional psychotherapy, expressive arts therapies, like art and play therapy, offer children non-verbal channels for expressing themselves.

In addition, both somatic experiencing and mindfulness practices are essential parts of holistic approaches. Somatic experiencing is concerned with the body's physiological reactions to trauma and aims to release stored tension; mindfulness, on the other hand, promotes present-moment awareness and helps children develop coping mechanisms and emotional regulation skills. Combining these various therapeutic modalities guarantees a thorough examination of the child's experiences and fosters a deeper comprehension of the complex interactions between psychological and physiological aspects of trauma.

Including family-based interventions is just as important in the holistic toolbox. Since families are seen as a microcosm of the child's world, family therapy and other interventions like it work to fortify family ties and provide a haven for the child to heal.

Teaching caregivers about trauma-informed parenting gives them the skills they need to build a secure attachment with their child, which helps the child recover and lessens the effects of trauma. Holistic approaches, then, encompass a wide range of therapeutic modalities that together address the various aspects of childhood trauma, recognizing the interdependence of the mind, body, and social environment.

The Way To Prolonged Recovery:

Starting down the path to long-term healing for traumatized children requires a nuanced understanding of the temporal and evolving nature of the healing process. Holistic approaches acknowledge that healing is not a linear journey but rather a dynamic process with unique trajectories for each child. A therapeutic alliance between the child and the mental health professional is essential to this path because traumatized children may be reluctant to share their deepest feelings and thoughts. Building trust becomes a cornerstone because it provides a safe and compassionate relationship on which the subsequent therapeutic interventions can be based.

The temporal dimension of therapeutic interventions becomes increasingly important as children move through the healing process. While short-term interventions may concentrate on immediate stabilization, crisis management, and symptom alleviation, they also often introduce cognitive restructuring and emotion regulation skills to provide the child with immediate coping mechanisms. The holistic approach acknowledges that true healing goes beyond symptom management, with long-term interventions going deeper into the trauma to reframe distorted cognitions and cultivate a deep sense of self-worth and resilience in the child.

Education and psychoeducation are essential components of the extended healing process. Giving kids age-appropriate knowledge about trauma, its impacts, and coping mechanisms helps make sense of their experiences. In addition, letting kids make decisions about their care gives them a sense of agency and encourages them to take an active role in their healing process. When kids get a better understanding of what they've gone through, they're better able to advocate for themselves and control their emotions.

Long-term healing also requires multidisciplinary work. School-based interventions, for example, are critical to children's academic and social development. Teachers with trauma-informed training can establish a secure and nurturing classroom, which helps the child adjust to school life. Working with community resources, like youth groups and organizations, expands the child's social support system. Holistic healing acknowledges the complex web of influences on a child's life and works to strengthen each strand to contribute to a more resilient and healed individual.

Fostering Children's Resilience:

Holistic approaches place a strong emphasis on building adaptive coping strategies and a strong sense of self in traumatized children.

Resilience is the capacity to overcome adversity; it is not a fixed quality; rather, it is a skill that can be developed. The goal of holistic interventions is to provide children with the tools they need to overcome obstacles and build an internal locus of control and self-efficacy.

Providing a safe and predictable environment is a critical component of resilience building; routine and consistency play a pivotal role in assisting children to regain a sense of security and stability. Schools that have been trauma-informed, for example, place a high value on fostering a nurturing environment that recognizes the special needs of children who have experienced trauma.

In these settings, teachers and caregivers work together to establish routines, expectations, and positive reinforcement that will serve as the foundation for the child's emotional stability.

Additionally, establishing social ties and supportive relationships is critical to building resilience. Community engagement programs, mentorship programs, and peer support groups give kids a chance to interact with others who may have gone through similar things.

Holistic approaches acknowledge the value of these relationships in terms of offering emotional support, lowering feelings of loneliness, and creating a sense of belonging. By fortifying social ties, kids form a support system that greatly enhances their emotional health.

Fostering emotional intelligence is an additional aspect of promoting resilience in kids. Holistic approaches integrate communication techniques, empathy building, and emotional regulation skills to improve kids' capacity to recognize, understand, and communicate their feelings. By giving kids these tools, holistic approaches hope to enable kids to deal with the emotional challenges of life and navigate the intricacies of interpersonal relationships.

CONCLUSION

A key element of holistic approaches to healing is supporting children's development of resilience in the wake of trauma. This includes building a therapeutic alliance, navigating the dynamic path to long-term healing, and cultivating a resilient mindset that gives kids the tools they need to face challenges head-on and overcome adversity. Holistic approaches support the holistic well-being of traumatized kids by recognizing their innate strengths and assisting them on their path toward resilience and healing.